ANTI-INFLAMMATORY DIET FOR HEALTHY LIFE

Improve Your Life Style And Feel Better Every Day With Easy And Healthy Recipes

Allison Mitchell

© **Copyright 2021 – Allison Mitchell - All Rights Reserved**

The content contained within this book may not be reproduced, duplicated or transmitted without direct written permission from the author or the publisher. Under no circumstances will any blame or legal responsibility be held against the publisher, or author, for any damages, reparation, or monetary loss due to the information contained within this book. Either directly or indirectly.

Legal Notice:

This book is copyright protected. This book is only for personal use. You cannot amend, distribute, sell, use, quote or paraphrase any part, or the content within this book, without the consent of the author or publisher.

Disclaimer Notice:

Please note the information contained within this document is for educational and entertainment purposes only. All effort has been executed to present accurate, up to date, and reliable, complete information. No warranties of any kind are declared or implied. Readers acknowledge that the author is not engaging in the rendering of legal, financial, medical or professional advice. The content within this book has been derived from various sources. Please consult a licensed professional before attempting any techniques outlined in this book.

By reading this document, the reader agrees that under no circumstances is the author responsible for any losses, direct or indirect, which are incurred as a result of the use of information contained within this document, including, but not limited to, - errors, omissions, or inaccuracies.

TABLE OF CONTENTS

INTRODUCTION 9
   SYMPTOMS OF INFLAMMATION 9
   FOODS TO EAT 11
   FOODS TO AVOID 12
BREAKFAST 15
   SPICY MARBLE EGGS 15
   NUTTY OATS PUDDING 16
   ALMOND PANCAKES WITH COCONUT FLAKES 17
   OAT PORRIDGE WITH CHERRY & COCONUT 18
   GINGERBREAD OATMEAL BREAKFAST 19
   APPLE, GINGER, AND RHUBARB MUFFINS 20
   ANTI-INFLAMMATORY BREAKFAST FRITTATA 21
   BREAKFAST SAUSAGE AND MUSHROOM CASSEROLE 22
   YUMMY STEAK MUFFINS 23
SNACKS , SIDES AND APPETIZERS 25
   CAULIFLOWER SNACKS 25
   CUCUMBER YOGURT 26
   HUMMUS DEVILED 27
   EGGS 28
   HUMMUS WITH CELERY 29
   KALE CHIPS 30
   FRESH STRAWBERRY SALSA 31
   RICE WITH PISTACHIOS 32
   ROASTED CURRIED CAULIFLOWER 33
   CARAMELIZED PEARS AND ONIONS 34
LUNCH 37
   CILANTRO-LIME CHICKEN DRUMSTICKS 37
   COCONUT-CURRY-CASHEW CHICKEN 38
   TURKEY & SWEET POTATO CHILI 39
   MOROCCAN TURKEY TAGINE 40
   TURKEY SLOPPY JOES 41
   NUT-CRUST TILAPIA WITH KALE 42

- WASABI SALMON BURGERS 43
- CITRUS & HERB SARDINES 44
- DARING SHARK STEAKS 45
- CAJUN CHICKEN & PRAWN 46

DINNER 49
- BEEF WITH ASPARAGUS & BELL PEPPER 49
- SPICED GROUND BEEF 50
- GROUND BEEF WITH CABBAGE 51
- ROASTED ROOT VEGETABLES 52
- STIR-FRIED BRUSSELS SPROUTS AND CARROTS 53
- CURRIED VEGGIES AND POACHED EGGS 54
- GROUND BEEF WITH VEGGIES 55
- GROUND BEEF WITH CASHEWS & VEGGIES 56
- GROUND BEEF WITH GREENS & TOMATOES 57
- BEEF & VEGGIES CHILI 58
- GROUND BEEF & VEGGIES CURRY 59

DESSERTS 61
- MINT CHOCOLATE CHIP ICE-CREAM 61
- FLOURLESS SWEET POTATO BROWNIES 62
- CARAMELIZED PEARS 63
- PALEO RASPBERRY CREAM PIE 64

DRINKS 67
- VANILLA AVOCADO SMOOTHIE 67
- TRIPLE FRUIT SMOOTHIE 68
- PEACH MAPLE SMOOTHIE 69
- PINK CALIFORNIA SMOOTHIE 70
- CARROT AND ORANGE TURMERIC DRINK 71

CONCLUSION 73

INTRODUCTION

The anti-inflammatory diet is not just for weight loss, although you may lose weight while on this diet. It is not a limited, three-week trek to push current inflammation from the body. It is not a false, quick leap to health. It provides a specific, fresh approach to your life: a way of life complete with all the nutrients and minerals, calories, and proteins that one needs to live well and happily. The anti-inflammatory diet components will help boost your overall health by providing the necessary nutrients and inflammation-fighting compounds to allow your body to heal itself and maintain proper balance. You will begin to notice changes in how you look and feel. You will have a sense of renewed energy. Your skin will take on an unmistakable healthy glow. Your body will be working correctly, producing new healthy cells and calming the chaos of inflammation within your system. To follow the anti-inflammatory diet and reap the health benefits, you must understand yourself.

Symptoms of Inflammation

The main signs of inflammation include; heat, redness, pain, swelling, and muscle-function loss. These symptoms depend on the inflamed body part and its cause. Some of the widespread signs of chronic inflammation are:

- Frequent infections
- Weight gain.
- Body pain.
- Insomnia
- Fatigue
- Mood disorders like anxiety and depression
- Gastrointestinal problems like diarrhea, constipation, and acid reflux disease.

The typical symptoms of inflammation rely on various inflammatory effect problems. When the body's defense mechanism which influences the skin activates, it causes rashes. When you are dealing with rheumatoid arthritis, it affects the joints. Most of the signs and symptoms experienced are fatigue, tingling, joint pains, stiffness, and swelling.

Similarly, when experiencing inflammatory bowel, it typically influences the digestive system. Its usual signs consist of bleeding ulcers, anemia, weight loss, bloating, pains, diarrhea, and stomach pains. With multiple sclerosis, the condition occurs on the myelin sheath, which covers the nerve cells. Its signs consist of problems when passing out stool, double vision, blurred eyesight, fatigue, and cognitive issues.

If you encounter any of the symptoms and health problems, you could be suffering from inflammation. Many people link it to joint pains like arthritis, which can be signaled by swelling and aches. The problem is related to health problems, not just swollen joints. Nevertheless, all soreness is not bad. For instance, acute inflammation is vital throughout recovery from a twisted and puffy ankle.

It is easy to detect Chronic inflammation signs and causes. Insomnia, genetic predisposition, food intake, and other individual habits can cause it. Similarly, inflammation resulting from allergic may also develop in your gut.

Below are some of the possibilities that you may be having it:

- If you always feel tired to the extent of not having enough sleep, not getting enough nap, or sleeping excessively.

- Do you experience time-to-time aches and pains? It may also signify that you have arthritis.

- Are you experiencing any pain in the gut or stomachache? The pain may create inflammation. Gut inflammation may also cause cramping, bloating, and loose stools.

- A swollen lymph node is another sign of inflammation. These nodes lie in the neck, armpits, and groin, which swell if there is a problem in your system. When you have a sore throat, your neck nodes lump because the body's defense system has sensed the condition. These lymph nodes react since the body is fighting the infection. The nodes reshape as you heal.

- Is your nose stuffed up? If indeed, maybe it is a symptom of irritating nasal tooth cavities.

- Sometimes, your epidermis may protrude because of internal inflammation.

Foods to Eat

If you already eat an appropriate healthy diet, you will have no trouble incorporating these foods into your meals. You may already be enjoying them and need a few tweaks to increase their presence in your meal planning. Some of the right foods that prevent and reduce chronic inflammation are as follows:

Omega 3 Fatty Acids

Omega 3 fatty acids are found in fish and fish oil. They calm the white blood cells and help them realize there is no danger of returning to dormancy. Wild salmon and other fish are good sources; It is recommended to eat them three times a week. Other foods rich in Omega 3s are flax meal and dry beans such as navy beans, kidney beans, and soybeans. An Omega3 supplement may be helpful if you are not able to ingest enough of these foods.

Fruits and Vegetables

Most fruits and vegetables are anti-inflammatory. They are naturally rich in antioxidants, carotenoids, lycopene, and magnesium. Dark green leafy vegetables and colorful fruits and berries do much to inhibit white blood cell activity.

Protective Oils and Fats

Yes, there are a few oils and fats that are good for chronic inflammation sufferers. They include coconut oil and extra virgin olive oil. Butter or cream is also acceptable to consume. Ghee, made from butter, is even better because it has the lactose and casein removed – the very ingredients cause so much trouble if you have lactose intolerance or wheat sensitivity.

Fiber

Fiber keeps waste moving through the body. Since the vast majority of our immune cells reside in the intestines, it is essential to keep your gut happy. If that doesn't provide enough fiber, feel free to take a fiber supplement.

Miscellaneous

Eat foods with spices and herbs instead of bad fats and unsafe oils. Spices like turmeric, cumin, cloves, ginger, and cinnamon can enhance white blood cells' calming. Herbs like fennel, rosemary, sage, and thyme also reduce inflammation while adding delicious new flavors to your food.

Fermented foods like sauerkraut, buttermilk, yogurt, and kimchi contain helpful bacteria that prevent inflammation.

Healthy snacks would include a limited amount of unsweetened, plain yogurt with fruit mixed in, celery, carrots, pistachios, almonds, walnuts, and other fruits and vegetables.

Foods to Avoid

While many foods should be included in your diet to aid in reducing chronic inflammation, there are also some foods that you must avoid to help keep the inflammation down.

Processed foods and sugars are two of the biggest culprits when it comes to inflammation in the western diet. Processed foods are highly refined, causing them to lose much of their natural fiber and nutrients. They are often high in omega 6, trans fats, and saturated fats, increasing inflammation.

Sugar is one of the worst offenders when it comes to increased inflammation. Not only does it hide in many foods, studies have found that it is also very addictive. Because of this, you should expect to go through a withdrawal phase when you remove it from your diet. It can often cause headaches, cravings, and sluggishness. Give yourself some time to allow your body to work through it. You don't have to remove natural sugars from your diet entirely, but you should work towards eating them a few times a week and at no more than one meal per day.

Most fried foods, especially deep-fried foods, should be avoided as well. Usually, they are cooked in processed oils or lard and are coated in a refined flour that promotes inflammation.

You will want to pay attention to foods known as nightshades. Nightshades can be anti-inflammatory, but some people are sensitive to them; if you find you seem to have more inflammation after consuming nightshade, you may want to begin to make substitutions in your recipes.

BREAKFAST

Spicy Marble Eggs

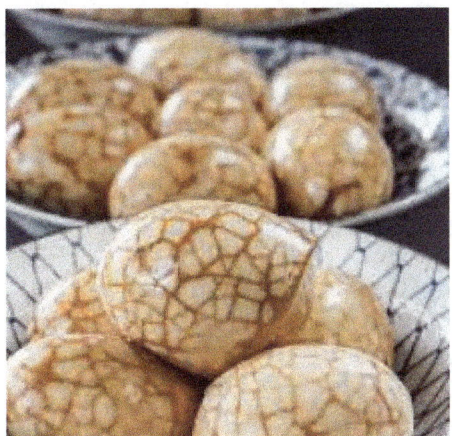

Preparation Time: 15 minutes - Cooking Time: 2 hours - Servings: 12

Ingredients:
6 medium-boiled eggs, unpeeled, cooled - For the Marinade - 2 oolong black tea bags
3 Tbsp. brown sugar - 1 thumb-sized fresh ginger, unpeeled, crushed - 3 dried star anise, whole
2 dried bay leaves - 3 Tbsp. light soy sauce - 4 Tbsp. dark soy sauce - 4 cups of water
1 dried cinnamon stick, whole - 1 tsp. salt - 1 tsp. dried Szechuan peppercorns

Directions:
Using the back of a metal spoon, crack eggshells in places to create a spider web effect. Do not peel.
Set aside until needed. Pour marinade into large Dutch oven set over high heat. Put lid partially on.
Bring water to a rolling boil, about 5 minutes. Turn off heat. Secure lid.
Steep ingredients for 10 minutes. Using a slotted spoon, fish out and discard solids.
Cool marinade completely to room proceeding.
Place eggs into an airtight non-reactive container just small enough to snugly fit all these in.
Pour in marinade. Eggs should be completely submerged in liquid. Discard leftover marinade, if any.
Line container rim with generous layers of saran wrap. Secure container lid.
Chill eggs for 24 hours before using. Extract eggs and drain each piece well before using, but keep the rest submerged in the marinade.

Nutrition:
Calories: 75 kcal - Protein: 4.05 g - Fat: 4.36 g - Carbohydrates: 4.83 g

Nutty Oats Pudding

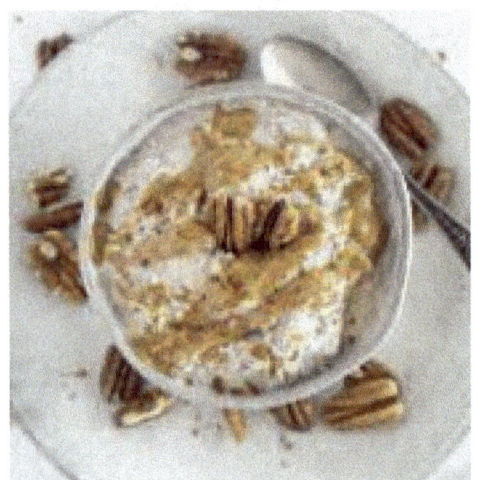

Preparation Time: 5 minutes - Cooking Time: 0 minutes - Servings: 3 -5

Ingredients:
¼ cup rolled oats
1 tablespoon yogurt, fat-free
1 ½ tablespoon natural peanut butter
¼ cup dry milk
1 teaspoon peanuts, finely chopped
½ cup of water

Directions:
Using a microwaveable-safe bowl, put together peanut butter and dry milk. Whisk well.
Add in water to achieve a smooth consistency. Add in oats.
Cover bowl with plastic wrap. Create a small hole for the steam to escape.
Place inside the microwave oven for 1 minute on high powder.
Continue heating, this time on medium power for 90 seconds. Let sit for 5 minutes.
To serve, spoon an equal amount of cereals in a bowl top with peanuts and yogurt.

Nutrition: Calories: 70 kcal - Protein: 4.25 g - Fat: 3.83 g - Carbohydrates: 6.78 g

Almond Pancakes with Coconut Flakes

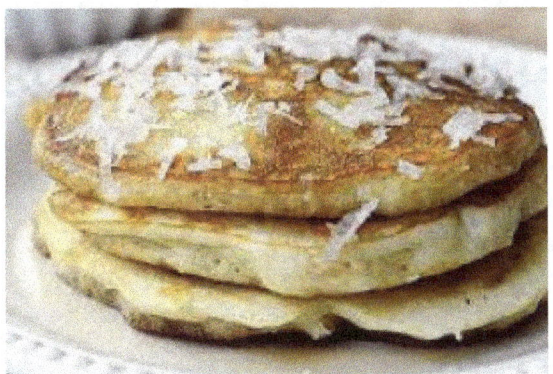

Preparation: Time: 5 minutes - Cooking Time: 10 minutes - Servings: 6

Ingredients:
1 overripe banana, mashed - 2 eggs, yolks, and whites separated - ½ cup unsweetened applesauce
1 cup almond flour, finely milled - ¼ cup of water - ¼ tsp. coconut oil - Garnish
2 Tbsp. blanched almond flakes - Dash of cinnamon powder - ¼ cup coconut flakes, sweetened
Pinch of sea salt - Pure maple syrup, use sparingly

Directions:
Whisk egg whites until soft peaks form. Except for egg whites and coconut oil, combine remaining ingredients in another bowl. Mix until batter comes together. Gently fold in egg whites. Make sure that you don't over mix, or the pancake will become dense and chewy. Pour oil into a nonstick skillet set over medium heat. Wait for the oil to heat up before dropping in approximately ½ cup of batter. Cook until each side are set, and bubbles form in the center. Turn on the other side then cook for another 2 minutes. Transfer flapjacks to a plate. Repeat step until all batter is cooked. Pour in more oil into the skillet only if needed. This recipe should yield between 4 to 6 medium-sized pancakes. Stack pancakes. Pour the desired amount of pure maple syrup on top. Garnish each stack with cinnamon-flavored almond-coconut flakes just before serving.

For the garnish, Set the oven to 350°F for at least 10 minutes before use. Line a baking sheet with parchment paper. Set aside. Mix almond and coconut flakes together in a bowl. Spread mixture evenly on a prepared baking sheet. Bake for 7 to 10 minutes until flakes turn golden brown. Stir almond and coconut flakes once midway through roasting to prevent over-browning. Remove the baking sheet from the oven. Cool almond and coconut flakes for at least 10 minutes before sprinkling in cinnamon powder and salt. Toss to combine. Set aside.

Nutrition: Calories: 62 kcal - Protein: 2.24 g - Fat: 4.01 g - Carbohydrates: 4.46 g

Oat Porridge with Cherry & Coconut

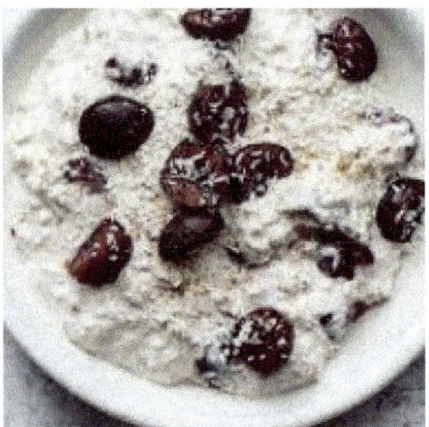

Preparation Time: 10 minutes - Cooking Time: 0 minutes - Servings: 3

Ingredients:
1 ½ cups regular oats - 3 cups coconut milk
4 tbsp. chia seed - 3 tbsp. raw cacao - Coconut shavings
Dark chocolate shavings - Fresh or frozen tart cherries
A pinch of stevia, optional - Maple syrup, to taste (optional)

Directions:
Combine the oats, milk, stevia, and cacao in a medium saucepan over medium heat and bring to a boil. Lower the heat, then simmer until the oats are cooked to desired doneness.
Divide the porridge among 3 serving bowls and top with dark chocolate and coconut shavings, cherries, and a little drizzle of maple syrup.

Nutrition:
Calories: 343 kcal - Protein: 15.64 g - Fat: 12.78 g - Carbohydrates: 41.63 g

Gingerbread Oatmeal Breakfast

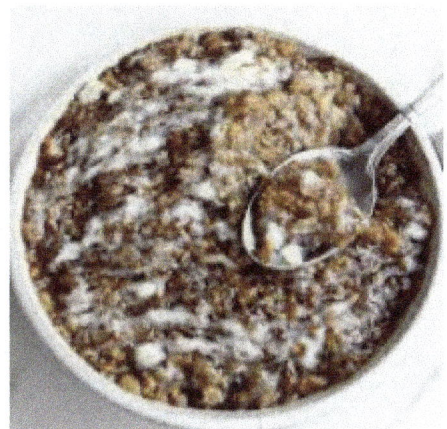

Preparation Time: 10 minutes - Cooking Time: 0 minutes - Servings: 4

Ingredients:
1 cup steel-cut oats - 4 cups drinking water
Organic Maple syrup, to taste - 1 tsp ground cloves
1 ½ tbsp. ground cinnamon - 1/8 tsp nutmeg
¼ tsp ground ginger - ¼ tsp ground coriander
¼ tsp ground allspice - ¼ tsp ground cardamom
Fresh mixed berries

Directions:
Cook the oats based on the package instructions. When it comes to a boil, reduce heat and simmer.
Stir in all the spices and continue cooking until cooked to desired doneness.
Serve in four serving bowls and drizzle with maple syrup and top with fresh berries.

Nutrition:
Calories: 87 kcal - Protein: 5.82 g - Fat: 3.26 g - Carbohydrates: 18.22 g

Apple, Ginger, and Rhubarb Muffins

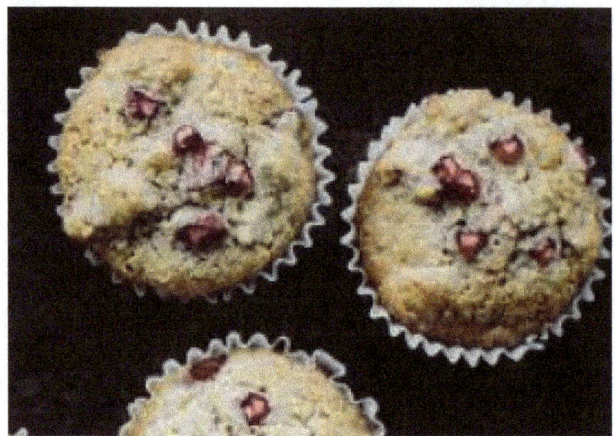

Preparation Time: 15 minutes - Cooking Time: 25 minutes - Servings: 4

Ingredients:

½ cup finely ground almonds - ¼ cup brown rice flour - ½ cup buckwheat flour
1/8 cup unrefined raw sugar - 2 tbsp. arrowroot flour - 1 tbsp. linseed meal
2 tbsp. crystallized ginger, finely chopped - ½ tsp. ground ginger
½ tsp. ground cinnamon - 2 tsp. gluten-free baking powder - A pinch of fine sea salt
1 small apple, peeled and finely diced - 1 cup finely chopped rhubarb
1/3 cup almond/ rice milk - 1 large egg - ¼ cup extra virgin olive oil - 1 tsp. pure vanilla extract

Directions:

Set your oven to 350F grease an eight-cup muffin tin and line with paper cases.
Combine the almond four, linseed meal, ginger and sugar in a mixing bowl.
Sieve this mixture over the other flours, spices and baking powder and use a whisk to combine well.
Stir in the apple and rhubarb in the flour mixture until evenly coated. In a separate bowl, whisk the milk, vanilla, and egg then pour it into the dry mixture. Stir until just combined – don't overwork the batter as this can yield very tough muffins.
Scoop the mixture into the arrange muffin tin and top with a few slices of rhubarb.
Bake for at least 25 minutes, till they start turning golden or when an inserted toothpick emerges clean. Take off from the oven and let sit for at least 5 minutes before transferring the muffins to a wire rack for further cooling. Serve warm with a glass of squeezed juice.

Nutrition: Calories: 325 kcal - Protein: 6.32 g - Fat: 9.82 g - Carbohydrates: 55.71 g

Anti-Inflammatory Breakfast Frittata

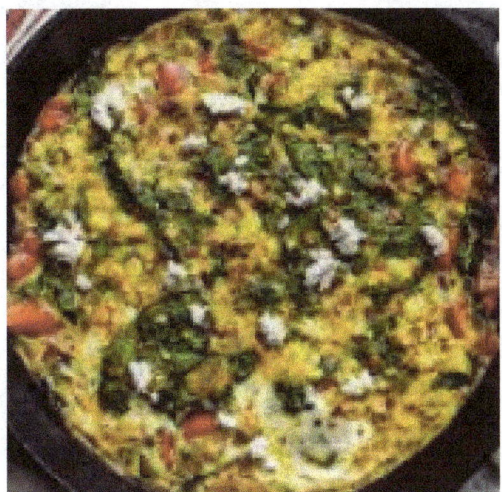

Preparation Time: 10 minutes - Cooking Time: 40 minutes - Servings: 4

Ingredients:
4 large eggs - 6 egg whites - 450g button mushrooms - 450g baby spinach
125g firm tofu - 1 onion, chopped - 1 tbsp. minced garlic - ½ tsp. ground turmeric
½ tsp. cracked black pepper - ¼ cup water - Kosher salt to taste

Directions:
Set your oven to 350F. Sauté the mushrooms in a little bit of extra virgin olive oil in a large non-stick ovenproof pan over medium heat.
Add the onions once the mushrooms start turning golden and cook for 3 minutes until the onions become soft. Stir in the garlic then cook for at least 30 seconds until fragrant before adding the spinach. Pour in water, cover, and cook until the spinach becomes wilted for about 2 minutes.
Take off the lid and continue cooking up to the water evaporates. Now, combine the eggs, egg whites, tofu, pepper, turmeric, and salt in a bowl.
When all the liquid has evaporated, pour in the egg mixture, let cook for about 2 minutes until the edges start setting, then transfer to the oven and bake for about 25 minutes or until cooked.
Take off from the oven then let sit for at least 5 minutes before cutting it into quarters and serving.
Baby spinach and mushrooms boost the nutrient profile of the eggs to provide you with amazing anti-inflammatory benefits.

Nutrition: Calories: 521 kcal - Protein: 29.13 g - Fat: 10.45 g - Carbohydrates: 94.94 g

Breakfast Sausage and Mushroom Casserole

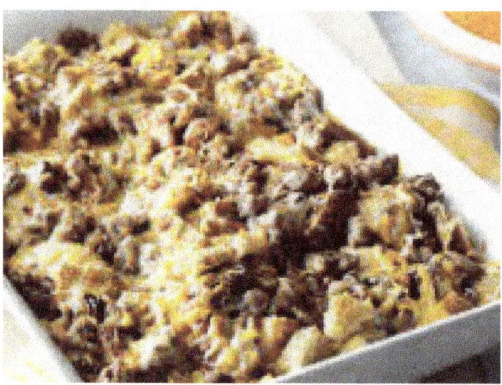

Preparation Time: 20 minutes - Cooking Time: 45 minutes - Servings: 4

Ingredients:
450g of Italian sausage, cooked and crumbled - Three-fourth cup of coconut milk
8 ounces of white mushrooms, sliced - 1 medium onion, finely diced
2 Tablespoons of organic ghee - 6 free-range eggs - 600g of sweet potatoes
1 red bell pepper, roasted - 3/4 tsp. of ground black pepper, divided - 1 ½ tsp. of sea salt, divided

Directions:
Peel and shred the sweet potatoes. Take a bowl, fill it with ice-cold water, and soak the sweet potatoes in it. Set aside. Peel the roasted bell pepper, remove its seeds and finely dice it. Set the oven 375°F. Get a casserole baking dish and grease it with the organic ghee. Put a skillet over medium flame and cook the mushrooms in it. Cook until the mushrooms are crispy and brown. Take the mushrooms out and mix them with the crumbled sausage. Now sauté the onions in the same skillet. Cook up to the onions are soft and golden. This should take about 4 – 5 minutes. Take the onions out and mix them in the sausage-mushroom mixture. Add the diced bell pepper to the same mixture. Mix well and set aside for a while. Now drain the soaked shredded potatoes, put them on a paper towel, and pat dry. Bring the sweet potatoes in a bowl and add about a teaspoon of salt and half a teaspoon of ground black pepper to it. Mix well and set aside. Now take a large bowl and crack the eggs in it. Break the eggs and then blend in the coconut milk.

Stir in the remaining black pepper and salt. Take the greased casserole dish and spread the seasoned sweet potatoes evenly in the base of the dish. Next, spread the sausage mixture evenly in the dish. Finally, spread the egg mixture. Now cover the casserole dish using a piece of aluminum foil.

Bake for 20 - 30 minutes. To check if the casserole is baked properly, insert a tester in the middle of the casserole, and it should come out clean. Uncover the casserole dish and bake it again, uncovered for 5 - 10 minutes, until the casserole is a little golden on the top. Allow it to cool for 10 minutes.

Nutrition: Calories: 598 kcal - Protein: 28.65 g - Fat: 36.75 g - Carbohydrates: 48.01 g

Yummy Steak Muffins

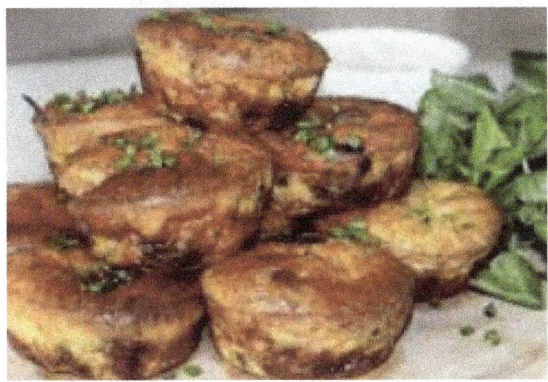

Preparation Time: 10 minutes - Cooking Time: 20 minutes - Servings: 4

Ingredients:
1 cup red bell pepper, diced
2 Tablespoons of water
8 ounce thin steak, cooked and finely chopped
¼ teaspoon of sea salt
Dash of freshly ground black pepper
8 free-range eggs
1 cup of finely diced onion

Directions:
Set the oven to 350°F. Take 8 muffin tins and line then with parchment paper liners.
Get a large bowl and crack all the eggs in it. Beat well the eggs. Blend in all the remaining ingredients. Spoon the batter into the arrange muffin tins. Fill three-fourth of each tin. Put the muffin tins in the preheated oven for about 20 minutes, until the muffins are baked and set in the middle.

Nutrition: Calories: 151 kcal - Protein: 17.92 g - Fat: 7.32 g - Carbohydrates: 3.75 g

SNACKS , SIDES AND APPETIZERS

Cauliflower Snacks

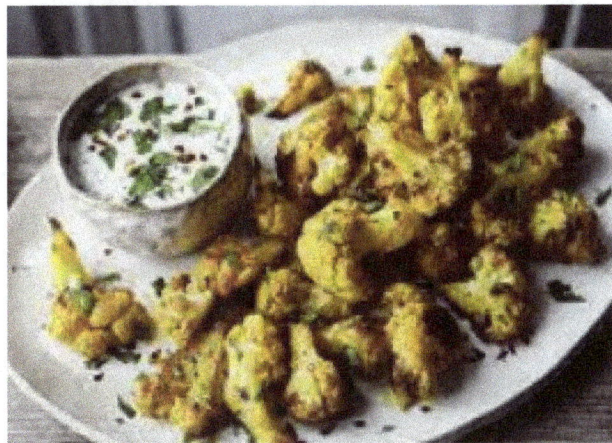

Preparation Time: 10 minutes - Cooking Time: 60 minutes - Servings: 4

Ingredients:
1 head of cauliflower
4 tablespoons extra virgin olive oil
1 teaspoon salt

Directions:
Set the oven to 425F, then prepare two cookie sheets by lining them with parchment paper.
Trim off the cauliflower florets and discard the core. Cut the florets into golf-ball-sized pieces.
Place the cauliflower in a bowl, and pour olive oil over them and sprinkle with salt.
Mix to coat. Spread in a single layer, not touching.
Roast about 1 hour, turning the cauliflower three to four times until golden brown.

Nutrition:
Calories: 91 kcal - Protein: 2.93 g - Fat: 7.7 g - Carbohydrates: 3.29 g

Cucumber Yogurt

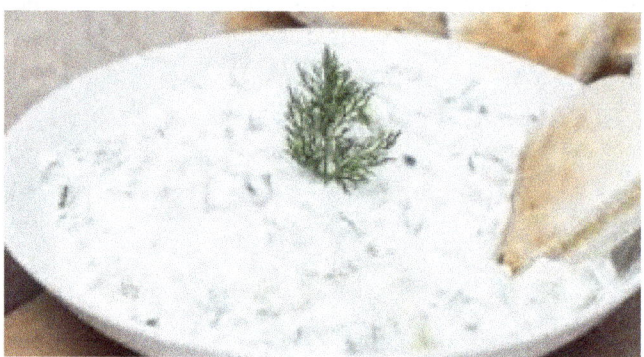

Preparation Time: 5 minutes - Cooking Time: 0 minutes - Servings: 1

Ingredients:
1 cup cucumbers, skin removed and chopped in chunks
2 tablespoons chopped cashews
1/4 cup fat-free Greek yogurt
2 teaspoons fresh-squeezed lemon juice
1 teaspoon fresh dill, chopped fine

Directions:
Peel and chop the cucumbers, then place them in a bowl.
Add the cashews, yogurt, lemon juice, and dill.
Mix well, grab a spoon, and enjoy.

Nutrition:
Calories: 300 kcal - Protein: 11.35 g - Fat: 23.55 g - Carbohydrates: 14.13 g

Hummus Deviled

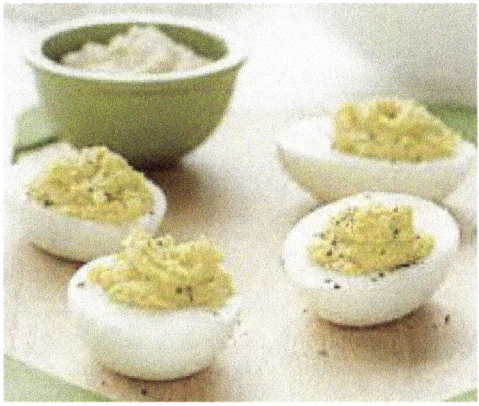

Preparation Time: 10 minutes - Cooking Time: 0 minutes - Servings: 6

Ingredients:
6 hard-boiled eggs
1/2 cup hummus
Paprika

Directions:
Slice the hardboiled eggs in half lengthwise and remove the yolk.
Fill the egg whites with hummus and sprinkle with paprika before serving.

Nutrition:
Calories: 179 kcal - Protein: 11.03 g - Fat: 12.41 g - Carbohydrates: 5.14 g

Eggs

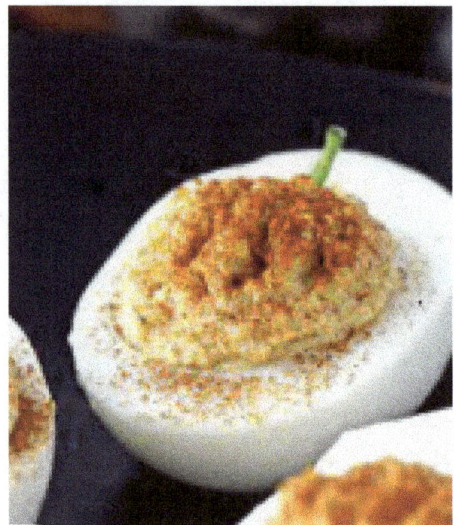

Preparation Time: 10 minutes - Cooking Time: 0 minutes - Servings: 6

Ingredients:
6 hard-boiled eggs
1/2 cup hummus
Paprika

Directions:
Slice the hardboiled eggs in half lengthwise and remove the yolk.

Fill the egg whites with hummus and sprinkle with paprika before serving.

Nutrition: Calories: 179 kcal - Protein: 11.03 g - Fat: 12.41 g - Carbohydrates: 5.14 g

Hummus with Celery

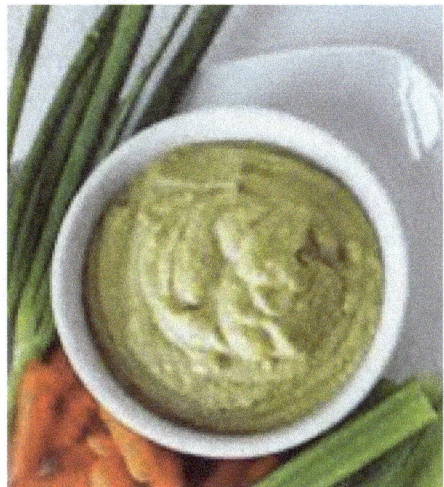

Preparation Time: 15 minutes - Cooking Time: 0 minutes - Servings: 4

Ingredients:
1/4 cup lemon juice - 1/4 cup tahini
3 cloves of garlic, crushed
2 tablespoons extra virgin olive oil
1/2 teaspoon salt - 1/2 teaspoon cumin
1 (15–ounce) can chickpeas
2 to 3 tablespoons water
Dash of paprika
6 stalks celery, cut into 2-inch pieces
3 tablespoons salsa

Directions:
Using a food processor mix the lemon juice and tahini for about a minute, until it is smooth.
Scrape the sides down and process for 30 more seconds. Add the garlic, olive oil, salt, and cumin.
Blend for about 1 minute. Drain the chickpeas, put the half of them on the food processor, and blend for another minute.
Scrape down the sides, add the other half of the chickpeas, and process until smooth, about 2 minutes.
If it like a little too thick, add water, 1 tablespoon at a time until you reach the desired consistency.
Fill the celery sticks with hummus and sprinkle paprika on top. Serve with salsa for dipping.

Nutrition: Calories: 240 kcal - Protein: 9.27 g - Fat: 14.51 g - Carbohydrates: 21.01 g

Kale Chips

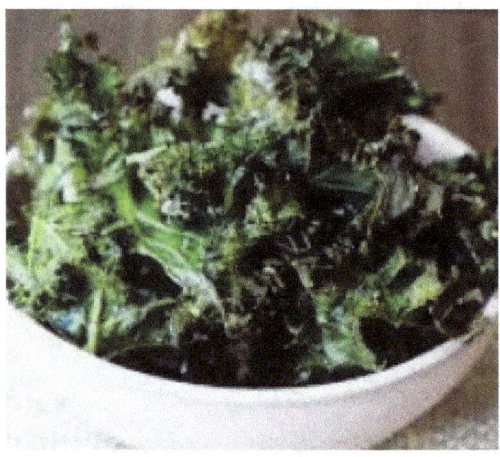

Preparation Time: 10 minutes - Cooking Time: 2 hours - Servings: 8

Ingredients:
2 bunches of curly kale with stems removed, washed and torn into bite-sized pieces
1 cup grated sweet potato
1 cup cashews, soaked and softened in water about 2 hours
2 tablespoons nutritional yeast (found at health food stores)
The juice of 1 lemon - 2 tablespoons honey
1/2 teaspoon sea salt - 2 tablespoons water

Directions:
Put the kale in a huge bowl and set aside. In a blender or food processor, process the sweet potato, softened cashews yeast, lemon juice, honey, salt, and water until smooth.
Put the mixture on the kale and toss with your hands to coat the leaves. Spread the kale leaves out on a large cookie sheet in a single layer without touching. Set the oven to its lowest setting.
Prop the oven door slightly ajar and dehydrate the chips for about 2 hours, turning the cookie sheet and watching to make sure the chips do not burn.
When crisp, remove from the oven and let cool. Store in an airtight container.

Nutrition: Calories: 40 kcal - Protein: 2.19 g - Fat: 0.87 g - Carbohydrates: 6.39 g

Fresh Strawberry Salsa

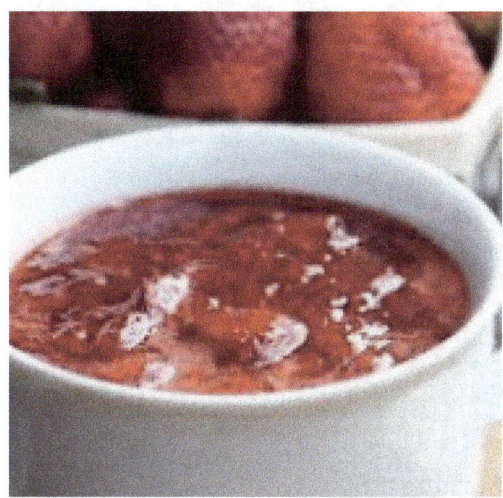

Preparation Time: 10 minutes - Cooking Time: 0 minutes - Servings: 6-8

Ingredients:
½ teaspoon lime zest, grated
2 teaspoons pure raw honey
2 kiwi fruit, peeled, chopped
½ cup fresh cilantro
¼ cup fresh lime juice
2 pounds fresh ripe strawberries, hulled, chopped
½ cup red onion, finely chopped
1-2 jalapeños, deseeded, finely chopped

Directions:
Add lime juice, lime zest and honey into a large bowl and whisk well.
Add rest of the ingredients then mix well.
Cover and set aside for a while for the flavors to set in. Serve.

Nutrition:
Calories: 119 kcal - Protein: 9.26 g - Fat: 4.38 g - Carbohydrates: 11.73 g

Rice with Pistachios

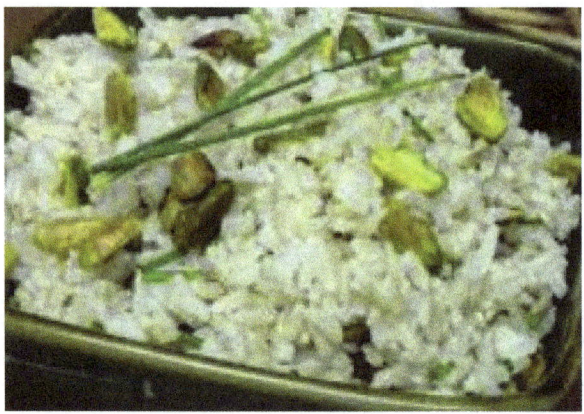

Preparation Time: 10 minutes - Cooking Time: 20 minutes - Servings: 6

Ingredients:
2 dry baby leaves - 1 thinly sliced medium onion - 5 pods of slightly crushed green cardamom
1 ½ cups of Basmati rice (rinsed in a colander and soaked in water for about 30 minutes, or more)
½ cup of chopped and packed dill leaves - ¼ cup of raw pistachios (or more for garnish)
3 cups of vegetable stock or water - ½ teaspoon of turmeric - 1 teaspoon of vegetable oil
Salt, to taste - Ground black pepper (to taste)

Directions:
In a large saucepan, warm the oil and add the cardamom.
Heat it for about 1 minute until it turns slightly brown and add the onion. Sauté for about 1-2 minutes.
Stir in the dill leaves, turmeric and pistachios. Then add the rice and stir-fry for about 1 minute.
Mix the vegetable stock, black pepper and salt to taste, stir it well and bring it to a boil.
Cover the pan using lid and cook over medium-low heat for about 15 minutes.
Take it off from the heat then set aside the rice (covered) for about 10 minutes.
Then fluff it with a fork and add more pistachios as garnish, if you desire.

Nutrition:
Calories: 90 kcal - Protein: 3.36 g - Fat: 5.08 g - Carbohydrates: 8.39 g

Roasted Curried Cauliflower

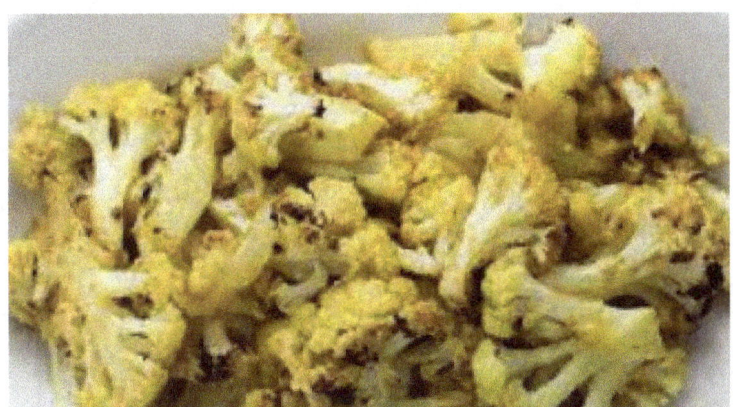

Preparation Time: 5 minutes - Cooking Time: 30 minutes - Serving: 4

Ingredients:
1 large head cauliflower, cut into florets
1 teaspoon curry powder
1 and ½ tablespoon olive oil
1 teaspoon cumin seeds
1 teaspoon mustard seeds
¾ teaspoon salt

Directions:
Preheat your oven to 375 degrees F
Grease a baking sheet with cooking spray. Take a bowl and place all ingredients. Toss to coat well. Arrange the vegetable on a baking sheet. Roast for 30 minutes

Nutrition: Calories: 67 - Fat: 6 g - Carbohydrates: 4 g - Protein: 2 g

Caramelized Pears and Onions

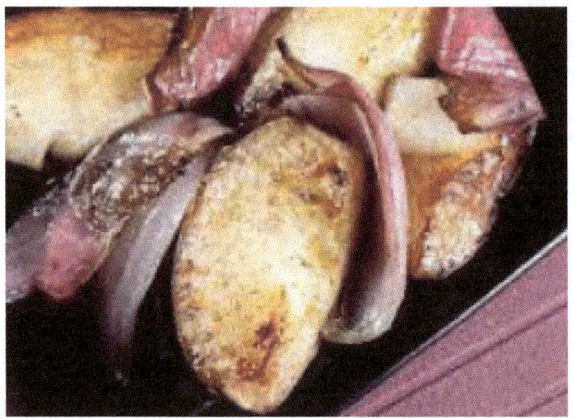

Preparation Time: 5 minutes - Cooking Time: 35 minutes - Serving: 4

Ingredients:
2 red onion, cut into wedges
2 firm red pears, cored and quartered
1 tablespoon olive oil
Salt and pepper, to taste

Directions:
Preheat your oven to 425 degrees F
Place the pears and onion on a baking tray, drizzle with olive oil, season with salt and pepper.
Bake in the oven for 35 minutes

Nutrition: Calories: 101 - Fat: 4 g - Carbohydrates: 17 g - Protein: 1 g

LUNCH

Cilantro-Lime Chicken Drumsticks

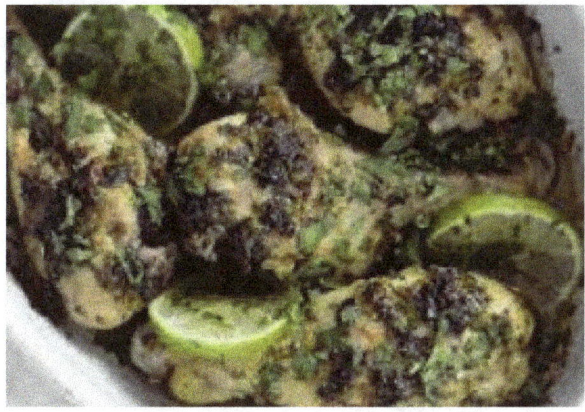

Preparation Time: 15 minutes
Cooking Time: 2 to 3 hours
Servings: 4

Ingredients:
¼ cup fresh cilantro, chopped - 3 tablespoons freshly squeezed lime juice
½ teaspoon garlic powder - ½ teaspoon sea salt
¼ teaspoon ground cumin - 3 pounds chicken drumsticks

Directions:
In a bowl, mix together the cilantro, lime juice, garlic powder, salt, and cumin to form a paste.
Put the drumsticks in the slow cooker. Spread the cilantro paste evenly on each drumstick.
Cover the cooker and set to high. Cook for 2 to 3 hours, or until the internal temperature of the chicken reaches 165°F on a meat thermometer and the juices run clear, and serve (see Tip).

Nutrition:
Calories: 417 - Total Fat: 12 g - Total Carbs: 1 g - Sugar: 1 g - Fiber: 1 g - Protein: 71 g - Sodium: 591 mg

Coconut-Curry-Cashew Chicken

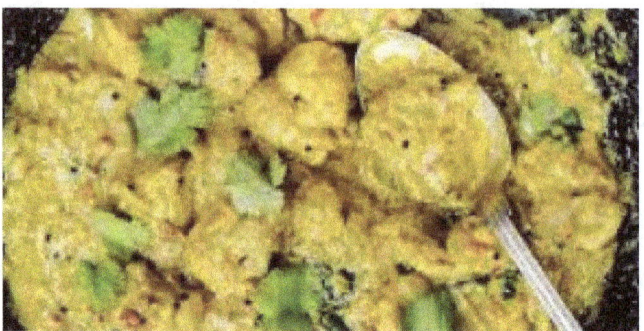

Preparation Time: 15 minutes - Cooking Time: 7 to 8 hours - Servings: 4

Ingredients:
1½ cups Chicken Bone Broth - 1 (14-ounce) can full-fat coconut milk
1 teaspoon garlic powder - 1 tablespoon red curry paste
1 teaspoon sea salt - ½ teaspoon freshly ground black pepper
½ teaspoon coconut sugar - 2 pounds boneless, skinless chicken breasts
1½ cup unsalted cashews - ½ cup diced white onion

Directions:
In a bowl, combine the broth, coconut milk, garlic powder, red curry paste, salt, pepper, and coconut sugar. Stir well. Put the chicken, cashews, and onion in the slow cooker.

Pour the coconut milk, mixture on top. Cover the cooker and set to low. Cook for around 7 to 8 hours, or until the internal temperature of the chicken reaches 165°F on a meat thermometer and the juices run clear. Shred the chicken using a fork, then mix it into the cooking liquid.

You can also remove the chicken from the broth and chop it with a knife into bite-size pieces before returning it to the slow cooker. Serve.

Nutrition:
Calories: 714 - Total Fat: 43g - Total Carbs: 21g - Sugar: 5g - Fiber: 3g - Protein: 57g - Sodium: 1,606mg

Turkey & Sweet Potato Chili

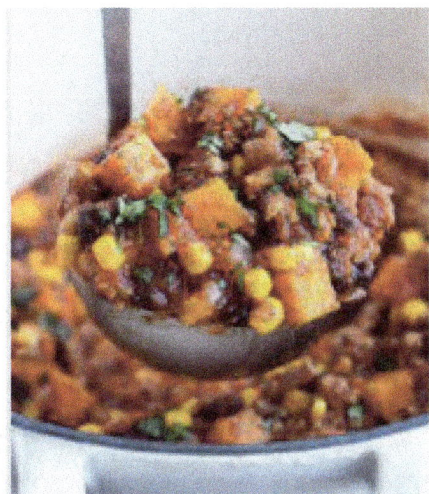

Preparation Time: 15 minutes - Cooking Time: 4 to 6 hours - Servings: 4

Ingredients:
1 tablespoon extra-virgin olive oil - 1 pound ground turkey
3 cups sweet potato cubes - 1 (28-ounce) can diced tomatoes
1 red bell pepper, diced - 1 (4-ounce) can Hatch green chiles
½ medium red onion, diced - 2 cups broth of choice
1 tablespoon freshly squeezed lime juice - 1 tablespoon chili powder
1 teaspoon garlic powder - 1 teaspoon cocoa powder
1 teaspoon ground cumin - 1 teaspoon sea salt
½ teaspoon ground cinnamon - Pinch cayenne pepper

Directions:
In your slow cooker, combine the olive oil, turkey, sweet potato cubes, tomatoes, bell pepper, chiles, onion, broth, lime juice, chili powder, garlic powder, cocoa powder, cumin, salt, cinnamon, and cayenne. Using a large spoon, break up the turkey into smaller chunks as it combines with the other ingredients. Cover the cooker and set to low. Cook for 4 to 6 hours. Stir the chili well, continuing to break up the rest of the turkey, and serve.

Nutrition:
Calories: 380 - Total Fat: 12g - Total Carbs: 38g - Sugar: 12g - Fiber: 6g - Protein: 30g - Sodium: 1,268mg

Moroccan Turkey Tagine

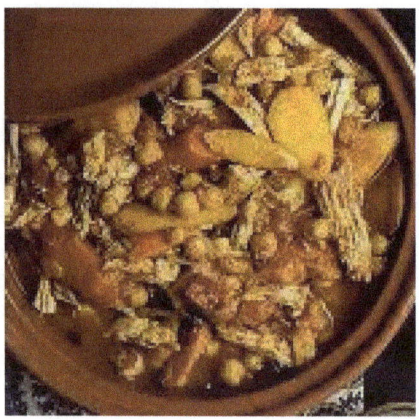

Preparation Time: 15 minutes - Cooking Time: 7 to 8 hours - Servings: 4

Ingredients:
4 cups boneless, skinless turkey breast chunks
1 (14 oz.) can diced tomatoes - 1 (14 oz.) can chickpeas, drained
2 large carrots, finely chopped - ½ cup dried apricots
½ red onion, chopped - 2 tablespoons raw honey
1 tablespoon tomato paste - 1 teaspoon garlic powder
1 teaspoon ground turmeric - ½ teaspoon sea salt
¼ teaspoon ground ginger - ¼ teaspoon ground coriander
¼ teaspoon paprika - ½ cup water
2 cups broth of choice - Freshly ground black pepper

Directions:
In your slow cooker, combine the turkey, tomatoes, chickpeas, carrots, apricots, onion, honey, tomato paste, garlic powder, turmeric, salt, ginger, coriander, paprika, water, and broth, and season with pepper. Gently stir to blend the ingredients.
Cover the cooker and set to low. Cook for 7 to 8 hours and serve.

Nutrition:
Calories: 428 - Total Fat: 5 g - Total Carbs: 46 g - Sugar: 25 g - Fiber: 8 g - Protein: 49 g - Sodium: 983mg

Turkey Sloppy Joes

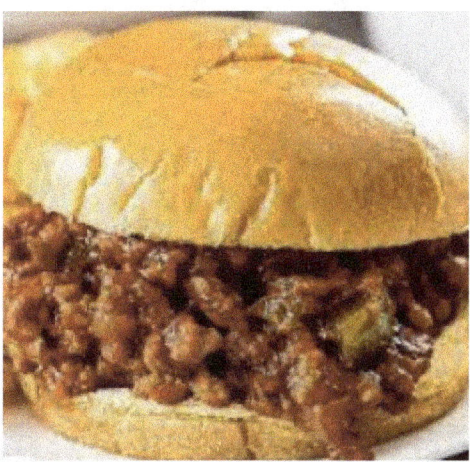

Preparation Time: 15 minutes - Cooking Time: 4 to 6 hours - Servings: 4

Ingredients:
1 tablespoon extra-virgin olive oil - 1 pound ground turkey
1 celery stalk, minced - 1 carrot, minced
½ medium sweet onion, diced - ½ red bell pepper, finely chopped
6 tablespoons tomato paste - 2 tablespoons apple cider vinegar
1 tablespoon maple syrup - 1 teaspoon Dijon mustard
1 teaspoon chili powder - ½ teaspoon garlic powder
½ teaspoon sea salt - ½ teaspoon dried oregano

Directions:
In your slow cooker, combine the olive oil, turkey, celery, carrot, onion, red bell pepper, tomato paste, vinegar, maple syrup, mustard, chili powder, garlic powder, salt, and oregano.
Using a large spoon, break up the turkey into smaller chunks as it combines with the other ingredients.
Cover the cooker and set to low. Cook for 4 to 6 hours, stir thoroughly and serve.

Nutrition:
Calories: 251 - Total Fat: 12 g - Total Carbs: 14 g - Sugar: 9 g - Fiber: 3 g - Protein: 24 g - Sodium: 690 mg

Nut-Crust Tilapia with Kale

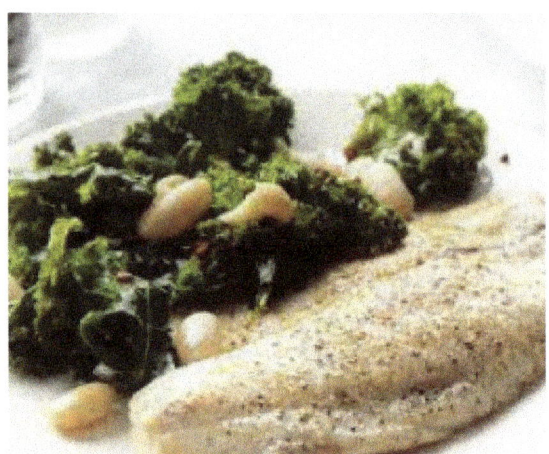

Preparation Time: 5 minutes - Cooking Time: 15 minutes - Servings: 2

Ingredients:
2 tsp. Extra virgin olive oil - 2 tbsp. Low-fat hard cheese, grated
1/2 cup Roasted and Ground Brazil Nuts/Hazelnuts/Any other hard nut
1/2 cup 100% Wholegrain breadcrumbs - 2 Tilapia Fillet, skinless
2 tsp. Whole grain mustard - 1 Head of kale, chopped
1 tbsp. Sesame seeds, lightly toasted -1 Garlic clove, minced

Directions:
Set the oven to 350°F. Lightly oil a baking sheet with the use of 1 tsp. extra virgin olive oil.
Mix in the nuts, breadcrumbs, and cheese in a separate bowl.
Spread a thin layer of the mustard over the fish and then dip into the breadcrumb mixture.
Transfer to baking dish. Bake for at least 12 minutes, till cooked through. Meanwhile, warm 1 tsp.
Oil in a skillet at medium heat temperature then sauté the garlic for 30 seconds, adding in the kale for a further 5 minutes. Mix in the sesame seeds. Serve the fish at once with the kale on the side.

Nutrition:
Calories: 475 kcal - Protein: 37.14 g - Fat: 33.44 g - Carbohydrates: 11.08 g

Wasabi Salmon Burgers

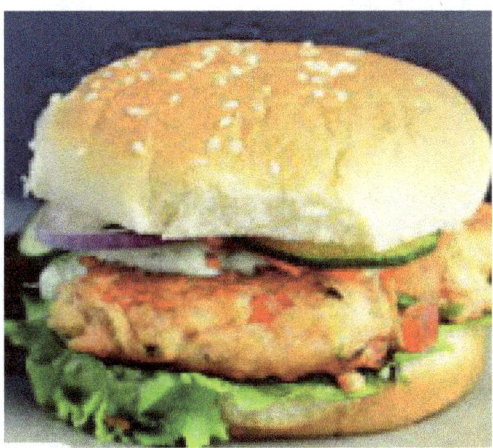

Preparation Time: 5 minutes - Cooking Time: 10 minutes - Servings: 1

Ingredients:
1/2 tsp. Honey
2 tbsp. Reduce-salt soy sauce
1 tsp. Wasabi powder
1 Beaten free-range egg
2 can Wild Salmon, drained
2 Scallion, chopped
2 tbsp. Coconut Oil
1 tbsp. Fresh ginger, minced

Directions:
Combine the salmon, egg, ginger, scallions, and 1 tbsp oil in a bowl, mixing well with your hands to form 4 patties. In a separate bowl, add the wasabi powder and soy sauce with the honey and whisk until blended. Heat 1 tbsp oil over medium heat in a skillet and cook the patties for 4 minutes each side until firm and browned. Glaze the top of each patty with the wasabi mixture and cook for another 15 seconds before you serve. Serve with your favorite side salad or vegetables for a healthy treat.

Nutrition: Calories: 591 kcal - Protein: 63.52 g - Fat: 34.3 g - Carbohydrates: 3.83 g

Citrus & Herb Sardines

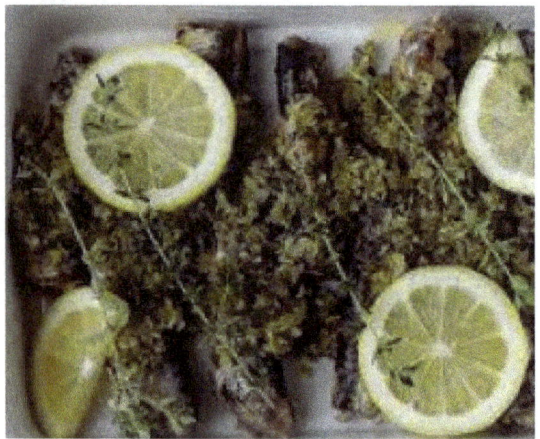

Preparation Time: 5 minutes Cooking Time: 15 minutes - Serv- ings: 2

Ingredients:
10 Sardines, scaled and clean - 2 Whole Lemon zest - Handful-Flat leafy parsley, chopped
2 Garlic cloves, finely chopped - 1/2 cup Black Olives (pitted and halves) - 3 tbsp. Olive oil
1 can Tomato, chopped, (optional) - 1/2 can Chickpeas or Butterbeans, drained and rinsed
8 Cherry Tomatoes, halved (optional) - Pinch of Black Pepper

Directions:
In a bowl, add the lemon zest to the chopped parsley (save a pinch for garnishing) and half of the chopped garlic, ready for later. Put a very large skillet on the hob and heat on high.
Now add the oil and once very hot, lay the sardines flat on the pan.
Sauté for 3 minutes until golden underneath and turn over to fry for another 3 minutes. Place onto a plate to rest. Sauté the remaining garlic (add another splash of oil if you need to) for 1 min until softened. Pour in the tin of chopped tomatoes, mix and let simmer for 4-5 minutes.
If you're avoiding tomatoes, just avoid this step and go straight to chickpeas.
Tip in the chickpeas or butter beans and fresh tomatoes and stir until heated through.
Here's when you add the sardines into the lemon and parsley dressing prepared earlier and add to the pan, cooking for a further 3-4 minutes.
Once heated through, serve with a pinch of parsley and remaining lemon zest to garnish.

Nutrition:
Calories: 493 kcal - Protein: 24.16 g - Fat: 35.67 g - Carbohydrates: 20.92 g

Daring Shark Steaks

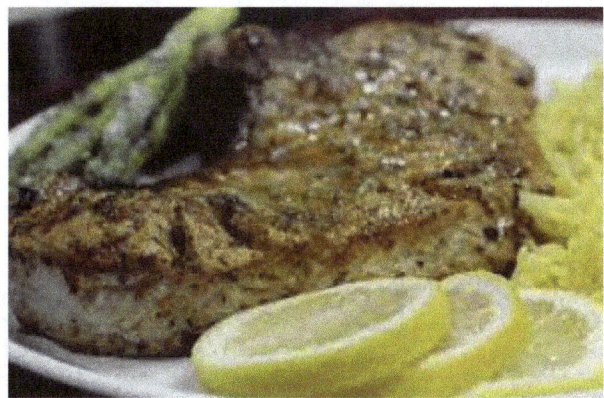

Preparation Time: 35 minutes - Cooking Time: 40 minutes - Servings: 2

Ingredients:
2 Shark steak, skinless
2 tbsp. Onion powder
2 tsp. Chili powder
1 Garlic clove, minced
¼ cup Worcestershire sauce
1 tbsp. Ground black pepper
2 tbsp. Thyme, chopped

Directions:
In a bowl, put then mix all of the seasonings and spices to form a paste before setting aside.
Spread a thin layer of paste on all sides of the fish, cover, and chill for 30 minutes (If possible).
Preheat oven to 325°F/150°C/Gas Mark 3.
Bake the fish in parchment paper for 30-40 minutes, until well cooked.
Serve on a bed of quinoa or whole-grain couscous and your favorite salad.

Nutrition: Calories: 112 kcal - Protein: 4.87 g - Fat: 3.65 g - Carbohydrates: 16.78 g

Cajun Chicken & Prawn

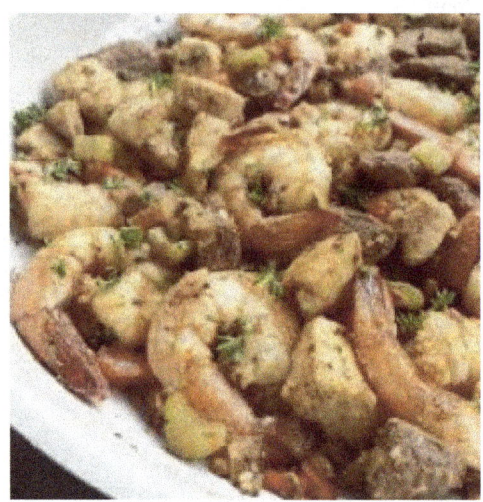

Preparation Time: 5 minutes - Cooking Time: 35 minutes - Servings: 2

Ingredients:
2 Free-range Skinless Chicken breast, chopped - 1 Onion, chopped
1 Red pepper, chopped - 2 Garlic cloves, crushed - 10 Fresh or frozen prawn
1 tsp. Cayenne powder - 1 tsp. Chili powder - 1 tsp. Paprika
1/4 tsp. Chili powder - 1 tsp. Dried oregano - 1 tsp. Dried thyme
1 cup Brown or wholegrain rice - 1 tbsp. Extra Virgin olive oil
1 can Tomatoes, chopped - 2 cups Homemade chicken stock

Directions:
In a bowl, put all the spices and herbs then mix to form your Cajun spice mix.
Grab a large pan and add the olive oil, heating on medium heat.
Add the chicken and brown each side for around 4-5 minutes. Place to one side.
Add the onion to the pan and fry until soft. Add the garlic, prawns, Cajun seasoning, and red pepper to the pan and cook for around 5 minutes or until prawns become opaque.
Add the brown rice along with the chopped tomatoes, chicken, and chicken stock to the pan.
Cover the pan and allow to simmer for around 25 minutes or until the rice is soft.

Nutrition:
Calories: 557 kcal - Protein: 18.96 g - Fat: 12.34 g - Carbohydrates: 93.28 g

DINNER

Beef with Asparagus & Bell Pepper

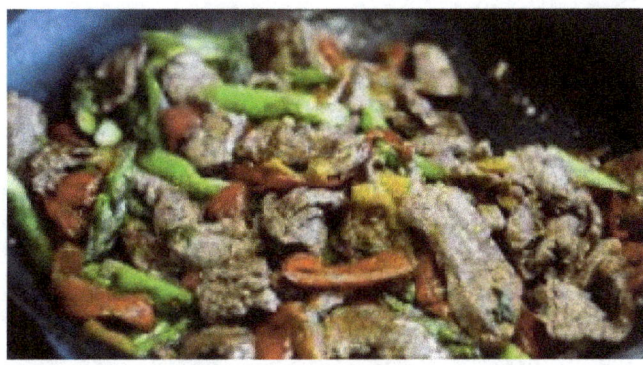

Preparation Time: 15 minutes - Cooking Time: 13 minutes - Servings: 4-5

Ingredients:
4 garlic cloves, minced - 3 tablespoons coconut aminos
1/8 teaspoon red pepper flakes, crushed - 1/8 teaspoon ground ginger
Freshly ground black pepper, to taste - 1 bunch asparagus, trimmed and halved
2 tablespoons olive oil, divided - 1-pound flank steak, trimmed and sliced thinly
1 red bell pepper, seeded and sliced - 3 tablespoons water - 2 teaspoons arrowroot powder

Directions:
In a bowl, mix together garlic, coconut aminos, red pepper flakes, crushed, ground ginger, and black pepper. Keep aside. In a pan of boiling water, cook asparagus for about 2 minutes.
Drain and rinse under cold water. In a substantial skillet, heat 1 tablespoon of oil on medium-high heat. Add beef and stir fry for around 3-4 minutes. With a slotted spoon, transfer the beef in a bowl.
In a similar skillet, heat remaining oil on medium heat.
Add asparagus and bell pepper and stir fry for approximately 2-3 minutes. Meanwhile, in the bowl, mix together water and arrowroot powder. Stir in beef, garlic mixture, and arrowroot mixture, and cook for around 3-4 minutes or till desired thickness.

Nutrition: Calories: 399 - Fat: 17 g - Carbohydrates: 27 g - Fiber: 8 g - Protein: 35 g

Spiced Ground Beef

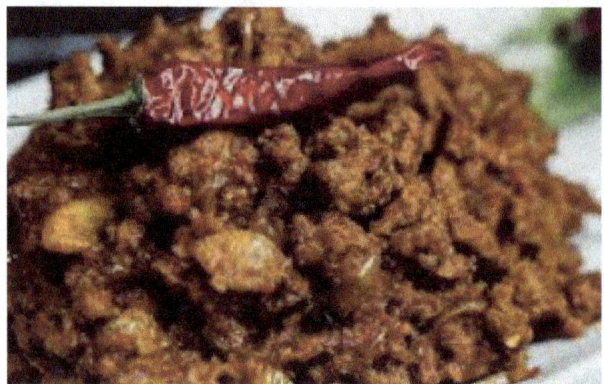

Preparation Time: 10 minutes - Cooking Time: 22 minutes - Servings: 5

Ingredients:
2 tablespoons coconut oil - 2 whole cloves - 2 whole cardamoms
1 (2-inch piece cinnamon stick - 2 bay leaves - 1 teaspoon cumin seeds
2 onions, chopped - Salt, to taste - ½ tablespoon garlic paste
½ tablespoon fresh ginger paste - 1-pound lean ground beef
1½ teaspoons fennel seeds powder - 1 teaspoon ground cumin
1½ teaspoons red chili powder - 1/8 teaspoon ground turmeric
Freshly ground black pepper, to taste - 1 cup coconut milk
¼ cup water - ¼ cup fresh cilantro, chopped

Directions:
In a sizable pan, heat oil on medium heat.
Add cloves, cardamoms, cinnamon stick, bay leaves, and cumin seeds and sauté for about 20-a few seconds. Add onion and 2 pinches of salt and sauté for about 3-4 minutes.
Add garlic-ginger paste and sauté for about 2 minutes. Add beef and cook for about 4-5 minutes, entering pieces using the spoon. Cover and cook approximately 5 minutes.
Stir in spices and cook, stirring for approximately 2-2½ minutes.
Stir in coconut milk and water and cook for about 7-8 minutes.
Season with salt and take away from heat. Serve hot using the garnishing of cilantro.

Nutrition: Calories: 444 - Fat: 15 g - Carbohydrates: 29 g - Fiber: 11 g - Protein: 39 g

Ground Beef with Cabbage

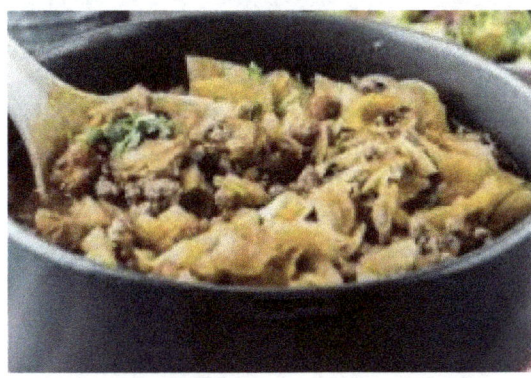

Preparation Time: 10 minutes - Cooking Time: 15 minutes - Servings: 6

Ingredients:
1 tbsp. olive oil - 1 onion, sliced thinly
2 teaspoons fresh ginger, minced
4 garlic cloves, minced
1-pound lean ground beef
1½ tablespoons fish sauce
2 tablespoons fresh lime juice
1 small head purple cabbage, shredded
2 tablespoons peanut butter
½ cup fresh cilantro, chopped

Directions:
In a huge skillet, warm oil on medium heat.
Add onion, ginger, and garlic and sauté for about 4-5 minutes.
Add beef and cook for approximately 7-8 minutes, getting into pieces using the spoon.
Drain off the extra liquid in the skillet. Stir in fish sauce and lime juice and cook for approx. 1 minute.
Add cabbage and cook approximately 4-5 minutes or till desired doneness.
Stir in peanut butter and cilantro and cook for about 1 minute. Serve hot.

Nutrition: Calories: 402 - Fat: 13 g - Carbohydrates: 21 g - Fiber: 10 g - Protein: 33 g

Roasted Root Vegetables

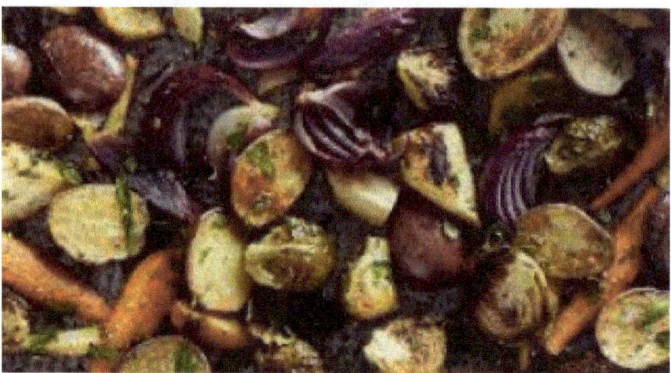

Preparation Time: 10 minutes - Cooking Time: 1 hour and 30 minutes - Servings: 6

Ingredients:
2 tbsp. olive oil - 1 head garlic, cloves separated and peeled
1 large turnip, peeled and cut into ½-inch pieces
1 medium-sized red onion, cut into ½-inch pieces
1 ½ lb. beets, trimmed but not peeled, scrubbed and cut into ½-inch pieces
1 ½ lb. Yukon gold potatoes, unpeeled, cut into ½-inch pieces
2 ½ lbs. butternut squash, peeled, seeded, cut into ½-inch pieces

Directions:
Grease 2 rimmed and large baking sheets. Preheat oven to 425oF.
In a huge bowl, mix all ingredients thoroughly.
Into the two baking sheets, evenly divide the root vegetables, spread in one layer.
Season generously with pepper and salt.
Place it into the oven, then roast for at least 1 hour and 15 minutes or until golden brown and tender.
Remove from the oven and let it cool for at least 15 minutes before serving.

Nutrition:
Calories 278 - Total Fat 5 g - Total Carbs 57 g - Net Carbs 47 g - Protein 6 g - Fiber 10 g - Sodium 124 mg

Stir-Fried Brussels Sprouts and Carrots

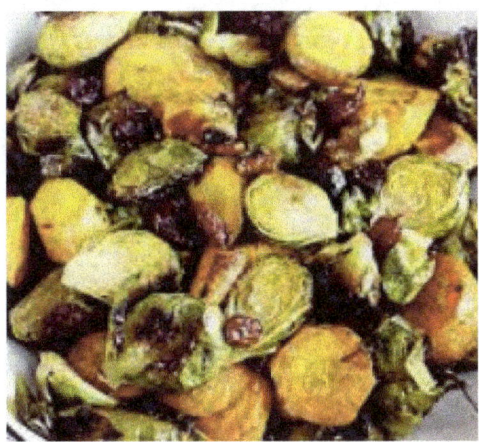

Preparation Time: 10 minutes - Cooking Time: 15 minutes - Servings: 6

Ingredients:
1 tbsp cider vinegar
1/3 cup water
1 lb. Brussels sprouts halved lengthwise
1 lb. carrots cut diagonally into ½-inch thick lengths
3 tbsp. olive oil, divided
2 tbsp. chopped shallot
½ tsp pepper ¾ tsp salt

Directions:
On medium-high fire, place a nonstick medium fry pan and heat 2 tbsp oil.
Ass shallots and cook until softened, around one to two minutes while occasionally stirring.
Add pepper salt, Brussels sprouts, and carrots.
Stir fry until vegetables start to brown on the edges, around 3 to 4 minutes. Add water, cook, and cover.
After 5 to 8 minutes, or when veggies are already soft, add remaining butter.
If needed, season with more pepper and salt to taste. Turn off fire, transfer to a platter, serve and enjoy.

Nutrition:
Calories 98 - Total Fat 4 g - Total Carbs 14 g - Net Carbs 9 g - Protein 3 g - Sugar: 5 g - Fiber 5 g

Curried Veggies and Poached Eggs

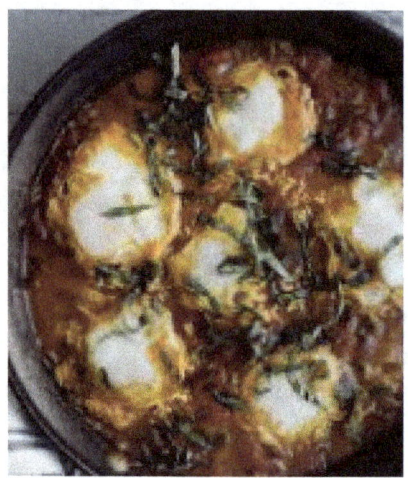

Preparation Time: 10 minutes - Cooking Time: 50 minutes - Servings: 4

Ingredients:
4 large eggs - ½ tsp white vinegar - 1/8 tsp crushed red pepper (optional)
1 cup water - 1 14-oz can chickpeas, drained - 2 medium zucchinis, diced
½ lb. sliced button mushrooms - 1 tbsp. yellow curry powder
2 cloves garlic, minced - 1 large onion, chopped - 2 tsp extra virgin olive oil

Directions:
On medium-high fire, place a large saucepan and heat oil. Sauté onions until tender around four to five minutes. Put the garlic and continue sautéing for another half minute. Add curry powder, stir and cook until fragrant around one to two minutes. Add mushrooms, mix, cover, and cook for 5 to 8 minutes or until mushrooms are tender and have released their liquid. Add red pepper if using, water, chickpeas, and zucchini. Mix well to combine and bring to a boil. Once boiling, reduce fire to a simmer, cover, and cook until zucchini is tender around 15 to 20 minutes of simmering.

Meanwhile, in a small pot filled with 3-inches deep water, bring to a boil on a high fire.

When boiling, lower the heat temperature to a simmer and add vinegar. Slowly add one egg, slipping it gently into the water. Allow to simmer until egg is cooked, around 3 to 5 minutes.

Take off the egg using a slotted spoon and transfer to a plate, one plate one egg. Repeat the process with remaining eggs. Once the veggies are done cooking, divide evenly into 4 servings and place one serving per plate of the egg. Serve and enjoy.

Nutrition: Calories 254 - Total Fat 9 g - Total Carbs 30 g - Net Carbs 21 g - Protein 16 g - Sugar: 7 g - Fiber 9g

Ground Beef with Veggies

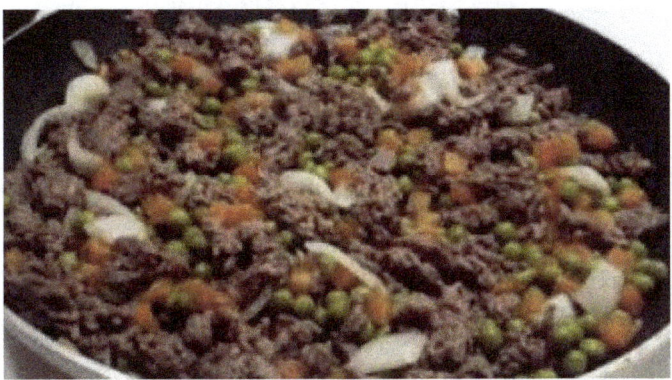

Preparation Time: 15 minutes - Cooking Time: 20 minutes - Servings: 2-4

Ingredients:
1-2 tablespoons coconut oil - 1 red onion, sliced
2 red jalapeño peppers, seeded and sliced
2 minced garlic cloves
1-pound lean ground beef
1 small head broccoli, chopped
½ of head cauliflower, chopped
3 carrots, peeled and sliced
3 celery ribs, sliced
Chopped fresh thyme, to taste
Dried sage, to taste - Ground turmeric, to taste
Salt, to taste - Freshly ground black pepper, to taste

Directions:
In a huge skillet, melt coconut oil on medium heat.
Add onion, jalapeño peppers and garlic and sauté for about 5 minutes.
Add beef and cook for around 4-5 minutes, entering pieces using the spoon.
Add remaining ingredients and cook, occasionally stirring for about 8-10 min.
Serve hot.

Nutrition: Calories: 453 - Fat: 17 g - Carbohydrates: 26 g - Fiber: 8 g - Protein: 35 g

Ground Beef with Cashews & Veggies

Preparation Time: 15 minutes
Cooking Time: 15 minutes
Servings: 4

Ingredients:

- 1½ pound lean ground beef
- 1 tablespoon garlic, minced
- 2 tablespoons fresh ginger, minced
- ¼ cup coconut aminos
- Salt, to taste
- Freshly ground black pepper, to taste
- 1 medium onion, sliced
- 1 can water chestnuts, drained and sliced
- 1 large green bell pepper, sliced
- ½ cup raw cashews, toasted

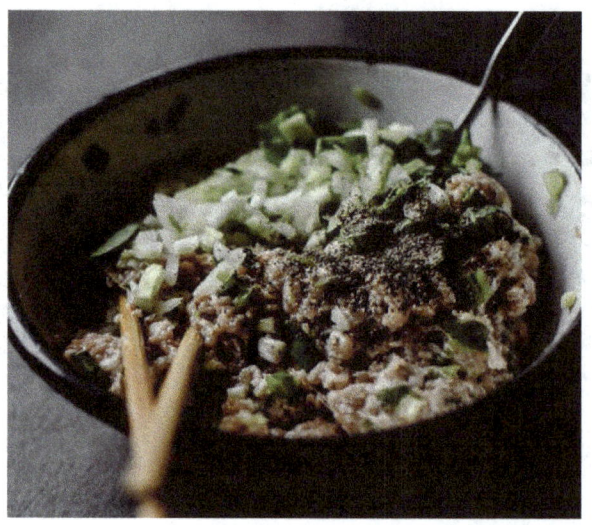

Directions:

Heat a nonstick skillet on medium-high heat. Add beef and cook for about 6-8 minutes, breaking into pieces with all the spoon. Add garlic, ginger, coconut aminos, salt, and black pepper and cook approximately 2 minutes. Put the vegetables and cook approximately 5 minutes or till desired doneness. Stir in cashews and immediately remove from heat. Serve hot.

Nutrition:

Calories: 452
Fat: 20 g
Carbohydrates: 26 g
Fiber: 9 g
Protein: 36 g

Ground Beef with Greens & Tomatoes

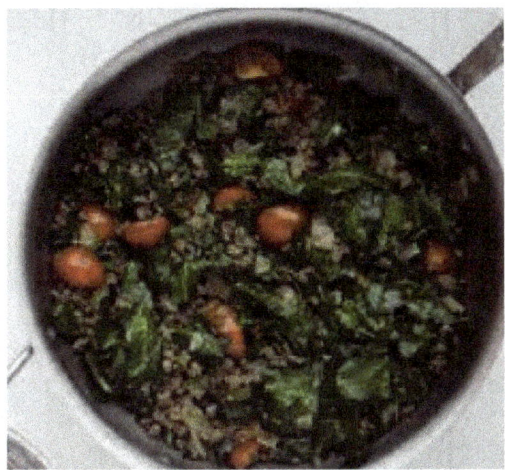

Preparation Time: 15 minutes - Cooking Time: 15 minutes - Servings: 4

Ingredients:
1 tbsp. organic olive oil - ½ of white onion, chopped
2 garlic cloves, chopped finely - 1 jalapeño pepper, chopped finely
1-pound lean ground beef - 1 teaspoon ground coriander
1 teaspoon ground cumin - ½ teaspoon ground turmeric
½ teaspoon ground ginger - ½ teaspoon ground cinnamon
½ teaspoon ground fennel seeds - Salt, to taste
Freshly ground black pepper, to taste - 8 fresh cherry tomatoes, quartered
8 collard greens leaves, stemmed and chopped - 1 teaspoon fresh lemon juice

Directions:
In a huge skillet, warm oil on medium heat. Put onion and sauté for approximately 4 minutes.
Add garlic and jalapeño pepper and sauté for approximately 1 minute.
Add beef and spices and cook approximately 6 minutes breaking into pieces while using spoon.
Stir in tomatoes and greens and cook, stirring gently for about 4 minutes.
Stir in lemon juice and take away from heat.

Nutrition:
Calories: 432 - Fat: 16 g - Carbohydrates: 27 g - Fiber: 12 g - Protein: 39 g

Beef & Veggies Chili

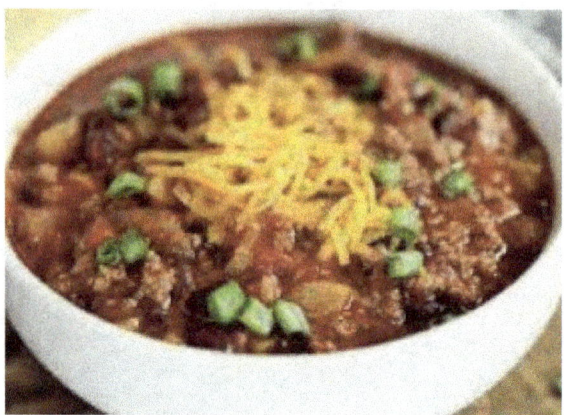

Preparation Time: 15 minutes - Cooking Time: 1 hour - Servings: 6-8

Ingredients:
2 pounds lean ground beef - ½ head cauliflower, chopped into large pieces
1 onion, chopped - 6 garlic cloves, minced - 2 cups pumpkin puree
1 teaspoon dried oregano, crushed - 1 teaspoon dried thyme, crushed
1 teaspoon ground cumin - 1 teaspoon ground turmeric
1-2 teaspoons chili powder - 1 teaspoon paprika - 1 teaspoon cayenne pepper
¼ teaspoon red pepper flakes, crushed
Salt, to taste Freshly ground black pepper, to taste
1 (26 oz.) can tomatoes, drained - ½ cup water - 1 cup beef broth

Directions:
Heat a substantial pan on medium-high heat. Add beef and stir fry for around 5 minutes.
Add cauliflower, onion, and garlic and stir fry for approximately 5 minutes.
Add spices and herbs and stir to mix well. Stir in remaining ingredients and provide to a boil.
Reduce heat to low and simmer, covered approximately 30-45 minutes. Serve hot.

Nutrition: Calories: 453 - Fat: 10 g - Carbohydrates: 20 g - Fiber: 8 g - Protein: 33 g

Ground Beef & Veggies Curry

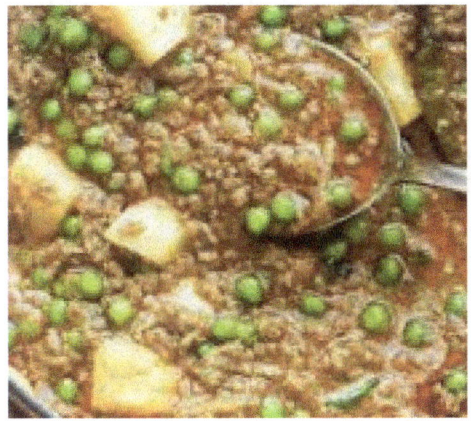

Preparation Time: 15 minutes - Cooking Time: 36 minutes - Servings: 6-8

Ingredients:
2-3 tablespoons coconut oil - 1 cup onion, chopped
1 garlic clove, minced - 1-pound lean ground beef
1½ tablespoons curry powder - 1/8 teaspoon ground ginger
1/8 teaspoon ground cinnamon - 1/8 teaspoon ground turmeric
Salt, to taste - 2½-3 cups tomatoes, chopped finely
2½-3 cups fresh peas shelled - 2 sweet potatoes, peeled and chopped

Directions:
In a sizable pan, melt coconut oil on medium heat.
Add onion and garlic and sauté for around 4-5 minutes.
Add beef and cook for about 4-5 minutes.
Add curry powder and spices and cook for about 1 minute.
Stir in tomatoes, peas, and sweet potato and bring to your gentle simmer.
Simmer covered approximately 25 minutes.

Nutrition: Calorie: 432 - Fat: 16 g - Carbohydrates: 21 g - Fiber: 11 g - Protein: 36 g

DESSERTS

Mint Chocolate Chip Ice-cream

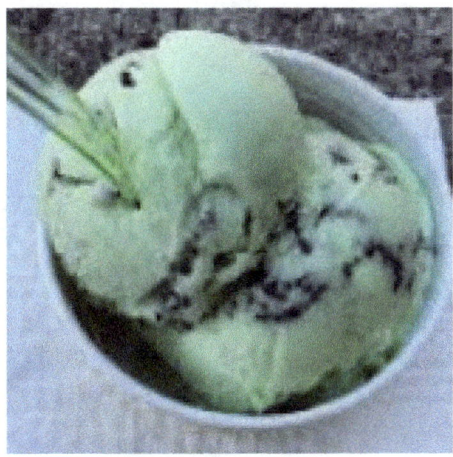

Preparation Time: 5 minutes - Cooking Time: 0 minutes - Servings: 2

Ingredients:
2 Frozen overripe bananas
Pinch Spirulina or any natural food coloring, optional.
3 tbsp. Chocolate chips or sugar-free chocolate chips
1/8 tsp. Pure peppermint extract - Pinch Salt
½ cup Raw cashews or coconut cream, optional.

Directions:
Mint or imitation peppermint won't be a substitute for this. Use pure peppermint extract and pour it all at once because a drop is more potent than you realize, so add slowly. Peel and cut the bananas first. Place the slices in a Ziplock bag then freeze. For the ice cream, put all the ingredients in a blender and pulse. You can skip the chocolate chips and just add them after blending. It'll turn out delicious either way. Serve as soon as it's ready or freeze until it's firm enough, then serve!

Nutrition: Calories: 250 kcal - Protein: 6.13 g - Fat: 24.37 g - Carbohydrates: 7.72 g

Flourless Sweet Potato Brownies

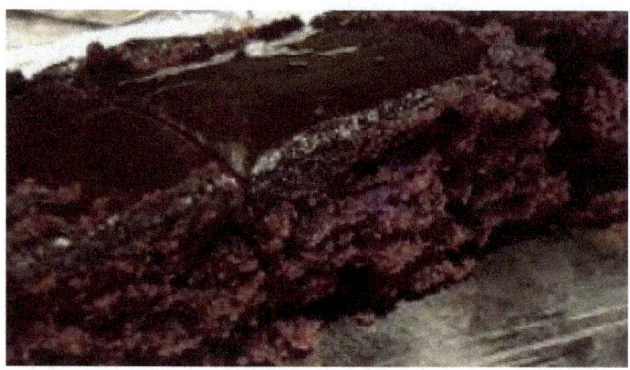

Preparation Time: 10 minutes - Cooking Time: 30 minutes - Servings: 9

Ingredients:
½ cup Cooked sweet potato - 2 tsp. Vanilla extract
½ cup Almond butter - 6 tbsp. Honey
½ tsp. Baking soda - 1 large Whole egg
¼ cup Unsweetened Cocoa powder
3 tbsp. Dairy-free chocolate chips, optional.

Directions:
Prep your oven by preheating to 350ºF. Line a baking pan with parchment paper leaving a few extra inches on the sides to make it easier to discard or remove. Blend all the ingredients, excluding the chocolate chips until you get a very smooth and soft batter. Transfer the creamy batter to your prepared baking pan and use a spatula to spread it around, so it looks almost even. Slide it in the oven, then bake for 30 minutes or until a knife inserted into the pan comes out clean. Take off from the oven and leave to cool in the pan for 15 minutes before putting it up on a wire rack.
If you decide to use the chocolate chip topping, put the chips in a microwave-safe dish and heat until it completely melts. Take off from the microwave and drizzle over the brownies.

Nutrition:
Calories: 171 kcal - Protein: 5.17 g - Fat: 9.28 g - Carbohydrates: 20.01 g

Caramelized Pears

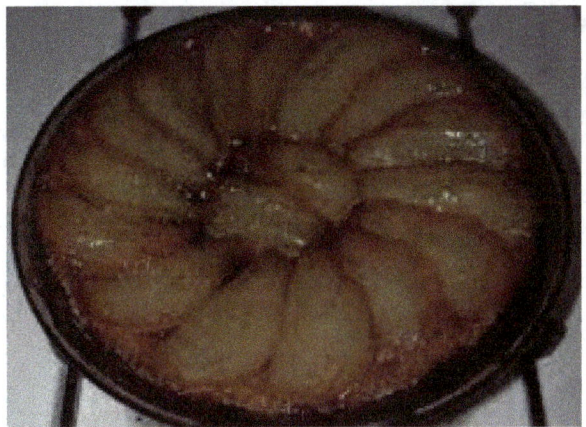

Preparation Time: 20 minutes - Cooking Time: 5 minutes - Servings: 5

Ingredients:
1 Teaspoon Cinnamon
2 Tablespoon Honey, Raw
1 Tablespoon Coconut Oil
4 Pears, Peeled, Cored & Quartered
2 Cups Yogurt, Plain
¼ Cup Toasted Pecans, Chopped
1/8 Teaspoon Sea Salt

Directions:
Get out a large skillet, and then heat the oil over medium-high heat.
Add in your honey, cinnamon, pears, and salt.
Cover, and allow it to cook for four to five minutes.
Stir occasionally, and your fruit should be tender.
Uncover it, and allow the sauce to simmer until it thickens.
This will take several minutes. Soon your yogurt into four dessert bowls.
Top with pears and pecans before serving.

Nutrition:
Calories: 290 - Protein: 12 g - Fat: 11 g - Carbs: 41 g

Paleo Raspberry Cream Pie

Preparation Time: 20 minutes - Cooking Time: 0 minutes - Servings: 12

Ingredients:
For the crust: 1 ½ tbsp. Maple syrup - Pinch Salt
½ cup Unsweetened shredded coconut - 1 tsp. Vanilla extract - 1 cup Roasted or salted cashews
Raspberry filling: ¾ cup Unrefined coconut oil - 1 ½ cup Roasted or salted cashews
½ cup & 1 tbsp. Maple syrup - ¼ cup & 2 tsp. Fresh lemon juice - ¼ cup Coconut cream from the top solid part of a can of coconut milk that has been refrigerated overnight - 2 tsp. Vanilla extract
3 cups Fresh raspberries - Pinch Salt

Directions:
Prepare 12 muffin pans, line them with muffin liners, and set them aside. Make the crust.
Set a pan over medium heat and the coconut and stir until it's completely toasted.
Stay by the pan because coconuts tend to burn very easily.
Transfer the toasted coconuts to a bowl and leave to cool for 5 minutes or so.
Honestly, this toasting step isn't particularly necessary, but I feel it adds amazing flavor to the crust.
To make the crust, put all the ingredients in a blender and pulse at the lowest speed until the mix gets all clumpy. Also, don't pulse for too long, or you might end up with a paste.
To know if it's ready, put a bit of the mixture on your fingers and pinch.
If it gets clumpy, you're on track, if not, add a little water and pulse at the lowest speed for further minutes. Scoop the mix into the lined tins using your fingers to pack the mix tightly inside the pan.
Put the pans to refrigerate while you get to make the filling.
In a tiny pot set over low heat, stir in all the ingredients until the oil and coconut cream melts completely. Clean the blender using a paper towel and pour in the filling.
Pulse at high-speed for like 60 seconds or until it's completely smooth.
The only clumps we can forgive are the raspberry seeds. Drizzle a quarter of the filling over the top of each crust. There should be extra filling; you can store and use that in another dish.
Place the coated muffins in the fridge to cool.
This will take a few hours, like 6 hours, so if you don't have time for that, put it in the freezer.
To serve, leave them to defrost for 80 minutes or until obviously creamy.

Nutrition:
Calories: 565 kcal - Protein: 7.74 g - Fat: 43.72 g - Carbohydrates: 42.72 g

DRINKS

Vanilla Avocado Smoothie

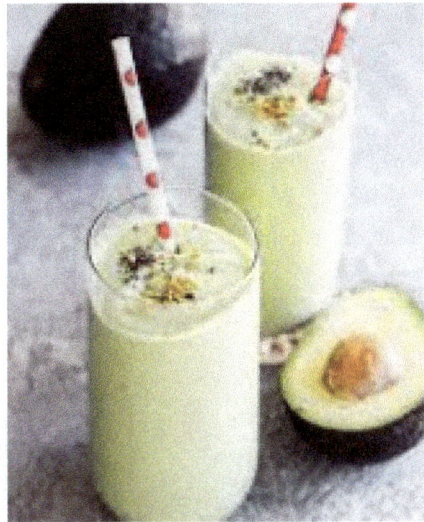

Preparation Time: 10 minutes - Cooking Time: 0 minutes - Servings: 1

Ingredients:
1 ripe avocado, halved and pitted
1 cup almond milk
1/2 cup vanilla yogurt
3 tbsp. honey
8 ice cubes

Directions:
Add everything to a blender jug. Cover the jug tightly. Blend until smooth.

Nutrition:
Calories: 143 - Fat: 1.2 g - Protein: 4.6 g - Carbs: 21 g - Fiber: 2.3 g

Triple Fruit Smoothie

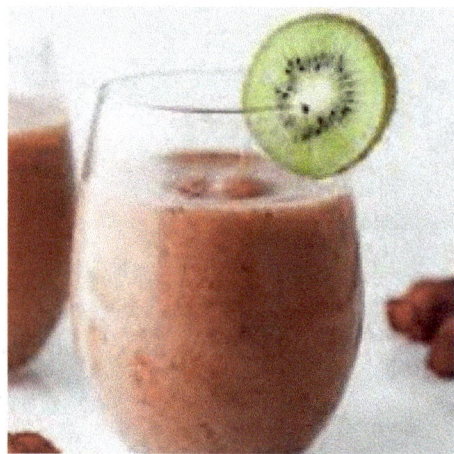

Preparation Time: 10 minutes - Cooking Time: 0 minutes - Servings: 1

Ingredients:
1 kiwi, sliced
1 banana, peeled and chopped
1/2 cup blueberries
1 cup strawberries
1 cup ice cubes
1/2 cup orange juice
1 container (8 oz.) peach yogurt

Directions:
Add everything to a blender jug. Cover the jug tightly. Blend until smooth.

Nutrition:
Calories: 124 - Fat: 0.4 g - Protein: 5.6 g - Carbs: 8 g - Fiber: 2.3 g

Peach Maple Smoothie

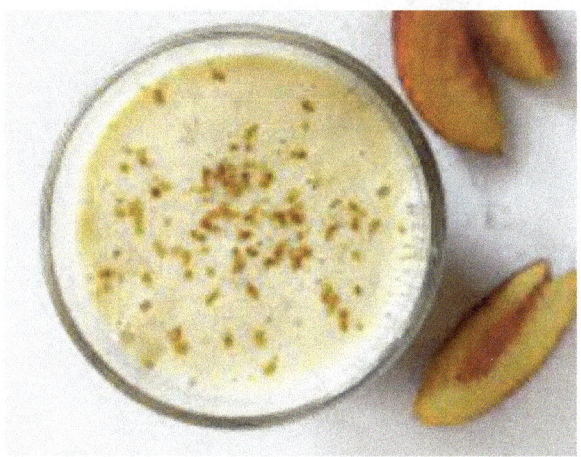

Preparation Time: 10 minutes - Cooking Time: 0 minutes - Servings: 1

Ingredients:
4 large peaches, peeled and chopped
2 tbsp. maple syrup
1 cup fat-free yogurt
1 cup ice

Directions:
Add everything to a blender jug. Cover the jug tightly. Blend until smooth.

Nutrition:
Calories: 125 - Fat: 0.4 g - Protein: 5.6 g - Carbs: 8 g - Fiber: 2.3 g

Pink California Smoothie

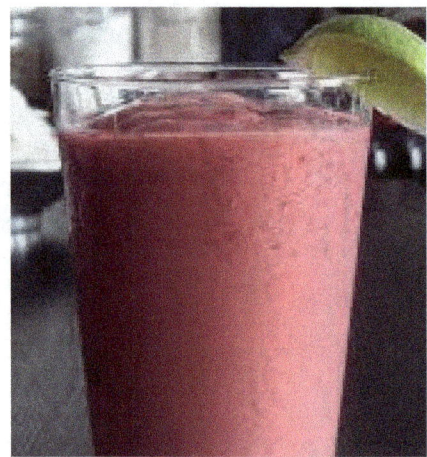

Preparation Time: 10 minutes - Cooking Time: 0 minutes - Servings: 1

Ingredients:
7 large strawberries
1 container (8 oz.) lemon yogurt
1/3 cup orange juice

Directions:
Add everything to a blender jug. Cover the jug tightly. Blend until smooth.

Nutrition:
Calories: 144 - Fat: 0.4 g - Protein: 5.6 g - Carbs: 8 g - Fiber: 2.3 g

Carrot and Orange Turmeric Drink

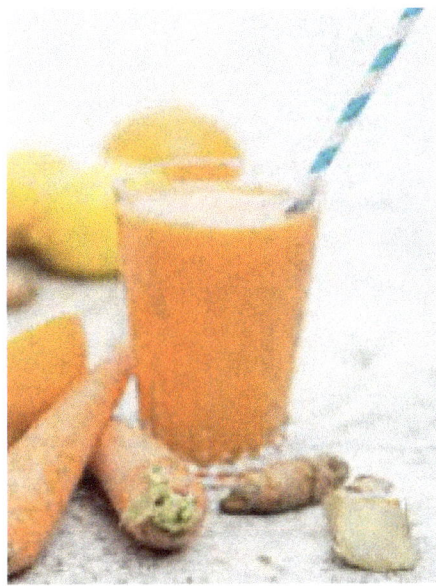

Preparation Time: 5 minutes - Cooking Time: 0 minutes - Servings: 2

Ingredients:
2 carrots, peeled, chopped
1 cup orange juice
1/2 inch ginger slice
2 tbsp. sugar
1 tbsp. lemon juice
1/4 tsp. turmeric powder

Directions:
In a blender, add orange juice, sugar, turmeric powder, carrots, and lemon juice. Blend well. Pour into serving glasses.

Nutrition:
Calories: 153 kcal -Protein: 4.47 g - Fat: 3.3 g - Carbohydrates: 27.02 g

CONCLUSION

Thank you for making it through to the end of the Anti-Inflammatory Diet Cookbook. Let's hope it was informative and able to provide you with all of the tools you must attain your goals, whatever they may be. Inflammation is a normal process of our immune system and completely necessary to protect us from threats that will damage our cells and tissues. If it weren't for our immune system, our bodies would be ravaged instantly by deadly diseases, and the results would be fatal. As long as the inflammatory process does not last beyond its normal time, there is usually no issue. Once the inflammation becomes chronic or long-term, it becomes an inflammatory disease and will create damaging results.

The inflammatory disease will lead to many different health consequences and will even attack our most vital organs. The best way to do this is to prevent chronic inflammation in the first place. The next best thing is to recognize the signs and symptoms as early as possible so that proper interventions can be done to limit and reverse the impact of chronic inflammation. Inflammatory disease is the root cause of many long-term diseases, so ignoring the warning signs can create major consequences for your health.

Unfortunately, if the inflammatory disease gets out of control, preventative measures may be out of the question, and medical interventions will need to be done. Our goal is to prevent you from getting to this point. Lucky for us, many lifestyle changes can be performed to stop and reverse this disease process when it is still in its advanced stages. This is another reason why we should recognize and not ignore the signs and symptoms. A major lifestyle change we can commit to is a new diet plan. The anti-inflammatory diet is a meal plan that boasts healthy and nutritious cuisines but still flavorful and appealing to the taste buds. There is a major myth out there that healthy food cannot be delicious. We have proven this myth wrong by providing numerous recipes worldwide that follow our healthy meal plan. We hope that the information you read in this book gives you a better understanding of how the immune system functions and how a proper diet plan can help protect it and our other valuable cells and tissues. The recipes we have provided are just a starting point. Use them as a guide to create many of your dishes that follow the diet plan. Just make sure you use the proper ingredients and food groups. Also, for maximum results, follow the Anti-Inflammatory Diet food guide.

The next step is to take the instruction we have provided and begin taking steps to change your life and improve your health. Begin recognizing the signs and symptoms of chronic inflammation and make the necessary lifestyle changes to prevent further health problems. Start transitioning to the anti-inflammatory diet today by incorporating small meals into your schedule and increase the amount as tolerated. Within a short period, the diet will be a regular part of your routine. You will notice increased energy, improved mental function, a stronger and well-balanced immune system, reduction in chronic pain, some healthy weight loss, and overall better health outcomes. If you are ready to experience these changes, then wait no longer and begin putting your knowledge from this book into action.

CPSIA information can be obtained
at www.ICGtesting.com
Printed in the USA
BVHW010852150621
609627BV00003B/263